Somatic exercises for weight loss 2024

Discover how to tap into your body's innate wisdom, Revolutionize your relationship with exercise and Restore balance, and Emotional Well being

Thomas P. Tinney

Copyright © [2024] by [Thomas P. Tinney]

This book is a work of non-fiction. All of the characters, incidents, and dialogue are drawn from the author's personal experiences, interviews, and research. Any resemblance to actual persons, living or dead, or events is entirely coincidental.

While the author has made every effort to provide accurate and up-to-date information, neither the author nor the publisher can be held responsible for any errors or omissions or for any consequences resulting from the use of this information.

Table of Contents

Chapter One: Introduction to Somatics and Weight Loss

1.1 Understanding Somatics' Role in Weight Management

The core of somatics resides in the complex web of human physiology, where the mind and body dance delicately together—a deep approach to understanding and utilizing the power of the mind-body connection. At its foundation, somatics goes deeply into sensory awareness, Movement, and perception, providing a comprehensive knowledge of how our physical and emotional experiences influence our overall wellbeing.

Somatics emerges as a light of insight and opportunity in weight control, providing a route to accessing the body's intrinsic intelligence and transformational potential. Unlike conventional techniques, which often concentrate on external issues such as nutrition and exercise, somatics pushes us to investigate the complex tapestry of sensations, emotions, and thinking patterns that impact our connection with food, Movement, and self-image.

Embodiment, or the process of living and completely experiencing our bodies in the present moment, is central to somatic practice. Through focused attention and bodily awareness, we may become more aware of the tiny subtleties of experience that develop inside us, such as the gradual rise and fall of the breath and the sensation of muscles engaging and releasing with each Movement.

As we expand our embodiment via somatic practices like breathwork, body scanning, and movement exploration, we develop a strong feeling of self-awareness and presence. We learn to listen to our bodies' signals, distinguishing between actual hunger and emotional needs, genuine exhaustion, and the urge to rest.

Furthermore, somatics provides a unique lens to explore the psychological and emotional aspects that lead to weight growth and weight control challenges. By investigating how previous experiences, traumas, and cultural pressures impact our relationship with food and our bodies, we gain insight into the underlying reasons for our difficulties. We may break free from the patterns that keep us stuck.

Crucially, somatics allows us to recover agency over our bodies and lives, enabling us to take an active role in our healing and change. Rather than considering weight reduction as a struggle to be fought or a goal to be met, somatics urge us to approach it as a journey of self-discovery and self-compassion—a journey led by inquiry, kindness, and a profound appreciation for the body's wisdom.

Understanding somatics in the context of weight control is embarking on a path of deep self-exploration and empowerment. It is to realize the interdependence of mind and body and to acknowledge that genuine change comes from a deeper relationship with oneself and a desire to accept the totality of our embodied experience rather than from external remedies or short fixes.

1.2 The Mind-Body Connection in Weight Loss.

Imagine yourself standing on the edge of a mountain, looking down over the great expanse of valleys below. As you breathe the fresh mountain air, tranquility washes over you, a deep connection between mind and body. This peaceful moment embodies the core of the mind-body connection—the dynamic interaction of our thoughts, emotions, feelings, and physical wellbeing.

Let us explore the complexities of this relationship further in the context of weight reduction. Consider the human body a highly tuned instrument, with each component contributing significantly to our life's symphony. The mind sits on the conductor's platform, arranging our everyday motions, rhythms, and melodies.

Regarding weight reduction, the mind significantly affects our habits, attitudes, and consequences. Consider how our ideas create our views and beliefs about ourselves and our bodies. If we hold self-limiting thoughts or engage in negative self-talk, we produce a dissonant note in the symphony of weight reduction, impeding progress and undermining our efforts.

In contrast, when we create a positive mindset of self-worth, resilience, and optimism, we tune our internal instrument to a harmonic song, propelling us ahead on our weight loss path with confidence and drive. It is the distinction between perceiving problems as impassable barriers and seeing them as chances for development and learning.

Emotions have an important part in the mind-body link. Consider the ebb and flow of emotion: waves slamming on the beach, stirring the core of our being. Stress, worry, and grief cause ripples in the fabric of our physiology, generating hormonal reactions that may alter our appetite, metabolism, and dietary preferences.

Consider the sense of hunger—a basic drive that arises in the stomach and the complicated network of neurons and neurotransmitters that make up our brain-gut connection. When we learn to listen to our bodies and distinguish between genuine hunger and emotional desires, we better understand our physical requirements and empower ourselves to make decisions that benefit our health and wellbeing.

Furthermore, the mind-body link goes beyond ideas and emotions, including the feelings and impulses inside our bodies. Techniques like mindfulness and somatic awareness help us tune in to our bodies' delicate rhythms and signals, guiding us toward choices that support our weight reduction objectives.

Imagine taking a deep breath, filling your lungs with air, and anchoring yourself in the present moment. That breath contains a moment of tremendous connection—a link between mind and body, thinking and feeling. It serves as a reminder that genuine change does not come from external solutions or fast fixes but from a growing understanding of ourselves and a commitment to interact with our inner terrain with curiosity, compassion, and bravery.

To summarize, the mind-body link in weight reduction is more than just a theoretical idea; it is a symphony of thoughts, emotions, experiences, and bodily sensations that weave together to form the song of our life. It is an invitation to deepen our connection with ourselves and our bodies, to listen to our inner knowledge, and to begin on a path of holistic healing and self-discovery.

1.3 How Somatic Exercises Can Help Weight Loss Goals

Close your eyes and envision yourself standing tall, planted like a strong oak tree, each breath flowing smoothly through your body. This visual vividly depicts the transformational impact of bodily exercises, which are dynamic approaches to Movement that improve the body and nourish the mind and soul. Let us take a voyage into the heart of somatics and see how it might guide the road to weight reduction success.

Somatics is an embodied awareness practice—an invitation to inhabit our bodies completely, listen to their messages, and move with purpose and grace. Unlike conventional forms of exercise, which often focus on external measurements like calories burnt or pounds lost, somatic exercises take a holistic approach that recognizes the interdependence of mind, body, and spirit.

Consider doing a sequence of mild motions that are fluid, flowing, and in sync with the rhythms of your breathing. These motions are more than simply a way to burn calories or shape muscles; they also provide a chance to develop a stronger feeling of self-awareness and presence. As you walk through each practice with attention and purpose, you unravel the layers of tension and stress that have built up inside your body, releasing them like autumn leaves blown away by the wind.

But somatic exercises give more than simply bodily relief; they also open the door to emotional healing and change. Imagine yourself doing a series of grounding exercises, sinking your roots into the soil and taking power and stability from the ground underneath you. You are exercising your body right now and reconnecting with your inner toughness and grit, building the framework for long-term transformation and progress.

Furthermore, somatic exercises provide a safe environment for self-expression and creativity, allowing you to explore movement patterns and feelings with curiosity and delight. Imagine doing a liberation dance, swaying, twisting, and spinning to the beat of your own heart. You are not constrained by norms or expectations in this moment of unrestricted mobility; you are free to express yourself completely, embracing the whole range of your nature.

Perhaps the most profound gift of somatic exercises is their potential to build a feeling of connectedness and compassion—for oneself, others, and the planet as a whole. Consider doing a series of heart-opening activities, such as extending your chest, raising your eyes to the sky, and connecting with the wealth of love and possibilities surrounding you. In this moment of vulnerability and openness, you understand that genuine change comes not from trying or struggling but from submitting to the body's wisdom and the flow of life.

To summarize, somatic exercises are more than simply a means to a goal; they are a journey of self-discovery, expression, and empowerment. They are an invitation to reclaim your body as a holy vehicle for development, change, and the journey of healing and wholeness. So, let us embrace the beauty of somatics and let it lead us on our journey to attain our weight reduction goals—not as a destination, but as an only dance of body, mind, and soul.

1.4 Advantages of Incorporating Somatics into Weight Loss Strategies

I. Improved Mind-Body Awareness.

- Greater awareness of physical feelings and emotions.
- Improved comprehension of the mind-body relationship in terms of eating habits and physical activity
- Increased capacity to distinguish between actual hunger and emotional desires.

II. Stress Reduction and Emotional Wellbeing

- Somatic activities improve relaxation and stress alleviation while lowering cortisol levels.
- Emotional healing via somatic activities, addressing underlying causes causing emotional eating.
- Cultivating self-compassion and acceptance while minimizing emotions of shame or guilt related to weight loss problems

III. Improved body image and self-esteem.

- Somatic activities promote a good connection with the body, emphasizing body awareness and acceptance.

- Individuals gain greater knowledge and respect for their body's potential, which increases their self-confidence.
- Shift from external validation to internal sources of self-worth, supporting lasting weight loss practices.

IV. Sustainable Weight Loss Strategies

- Somatic exercises stress comprehensive weight reduction treatments, concentrating on long-term health and wellbeing.
- Developing intuitive eating abilities allows people to make better meal choices based on internal indications.
- Incorporating mindful movement activities into everyday routines promotes regular physical exercise without fatigue.

V. Prevention of Weight Cycling and Yo-Yo Diets

- Somatic techniques target the underlying habits and behaviors that lead to weight swings.
- The emphasis on self-care and self-awareness decreases the chance of participating in excessive diets or restrictive eating behaviors.
- Promote a balanced approach to weight management, creating long-term habits for maintaining a healthy weight.

VI. A Holistic Approach to Wellness

- Integrating somatic exercises into general wellness practices to promote not just physical health but also mental and emotional wellbeing.
- Creating a conducive atmosphere for holistic health and personal development
- Empowering people to take ownership of their health and live fulfilled lives beyond weight loss objectives

1.5 Overcoming Obstacles and Myths in Somatic Weight Loss

The route to actual change is obscured by a labyrinth of hurdles and misconceptions in the quest for somatic weight reduction. However, with clarity and awareness, we may overcome these beliefs and emerge stronger, more resilient, and more in touch with our bodies' knowledge.

Imagine yourself at the start of your weight reduction journey, enthusiastic and motivated to go on a road of self-discovery and rebirth. However, when you take your initial steps, you get entangled in a web of doubt and confusion, with myths and misunderstandings whispering in your ear, threatening to derail your progress.

One of the most common misconceptions about somatic weight reduction is that it is a fast fix—a shortcut to dropping pounds without addressing the underlying causes that cause weight gain. This misconception, propagated by fad diets and magical cures, contradicts the holistic character of somatic practices, emphasizing the necessity of treating the mind-body link and developing long-term habits.

Another obstacle that people may face on their somatic weight reduction journey is the conviction that their bodies are intrinsically imperfect or unfit based on social norms of beauty and perfection. This perspective may create a barrier to self-acceptance and self-compassion, preventing people from fully embracing the transforming power of somatic practices.

Furthermore, there may be a misperception that somatic exercises are only appropriate for those who are already fit or flexible, eliminating those who are new to exercise or have physical restrictions. In actuality, somatic practices may be tailored to people of different ages, abilities, and fitness levels, providing a gentle yet effective approach to Movement and self-care.

Despite these problems and misconceptions, there is a beacon of hope—a guiding light that lights the route ahead. It is the knowledge that genuine change does not come from external solutions or fast fixes but rather from a growing awareness of ourselves and a desire to connect with our bodies and experiences with curiosity, compassion, and bravery.

By tackling the problems and removing the beliefs that stand in our way, we allow ourselves to experience deep healing and progress. We value our bodies' natural knowledge and recognize the interdependence of mind, body, and spirit. In doing so, we learn that the fundamental meaning of somatic weight reduction is not hitting a certain number on the scale but rather recovering our power, energy, and intrinsic value as human beings.

Challenge the Quick Fix Mentality:

- I was addressing the idea that somatic weight reduction is a fast remedy.
- I emphasize the integrative nature of somatic techniques and the significance of treating root causes.

Cultivating self-acceptance and compassion:

- We are overcoming the assumption that our bodies are fundamentally defective or inadequate.
- Encourage self-acceptance and self-compassion as essential components of somatic weight reduction.

Making Somatic Practices Inclusive.

- They are dispelling the idea that bodily exercises are intended for those already fit and flexible.
- I emphasize the flexibility of somatic activities to people of diverse ages, skills, and fitness levels.

Embracing Sustainable Habits

- They reject the myth that somatic weight reduction necessitates drastic or unsustainable tactics.
- For long-term outcomes, encourage the development of durable habits and lifestyle modifications.

Prioritizing the Mind-Body Connection:

- Recognize the significance of the mind-body relationship in somatic weight reduction.
- Encourage activities that promote mindfulness, self-awareness, and emotional wellbeing in addition to physical exercise.

Chapter 2: The Foundations of Somatic Exercise

2.1 Breathwork Techniques for Somatic Awareness.

Breathwork is a core technique in somatic awareness, working as a link between the mind and body and allowing us to connect more deeply with our inner environment. Below, we will look at numerous breathwork methods and provide detailed examples to help you understand and practice them.

Diaphragmatic Breath:

Technique:

- Sit or lay comfortably with one hand on your chest and the other on your belly.
- Inhale deeply through your nose, feeling your belly rise as you fill your lungs with air.
- Exhale gently through your lips, feeling your stomach drop.

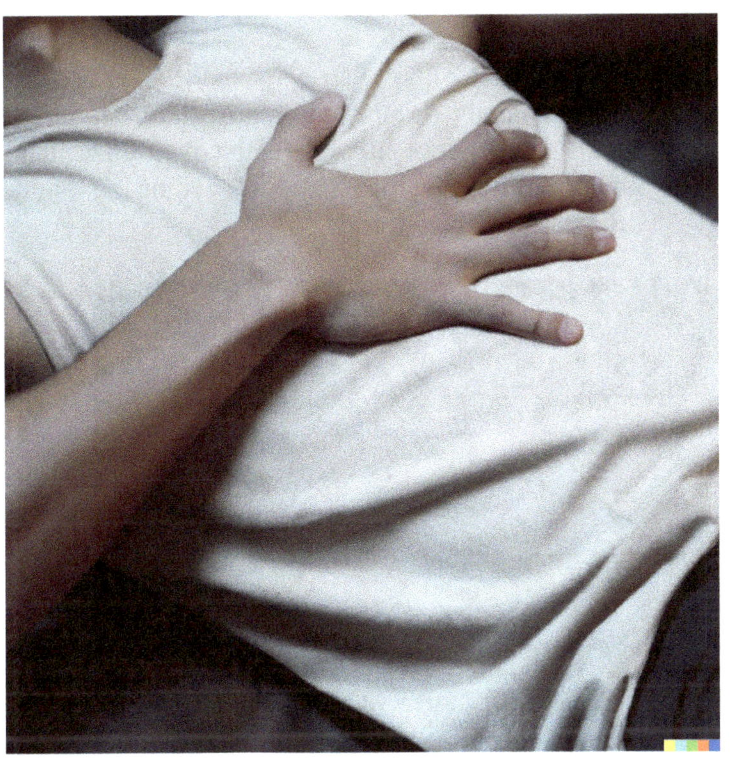

Box breathing (or square breathing):

- Inhale deeply through your nose for a count of four. Hold your breath for a count of four. Exhale gently through your lips for a count of four. Hold your breath for a count of four before starting the following cycle.

Breathing: 4-7-8

- Inhale deeply through your nose for a count of four. Hold your breath for a count of seven. Exhale gently through your lips for a count of eight. Repeat for a few rounds.

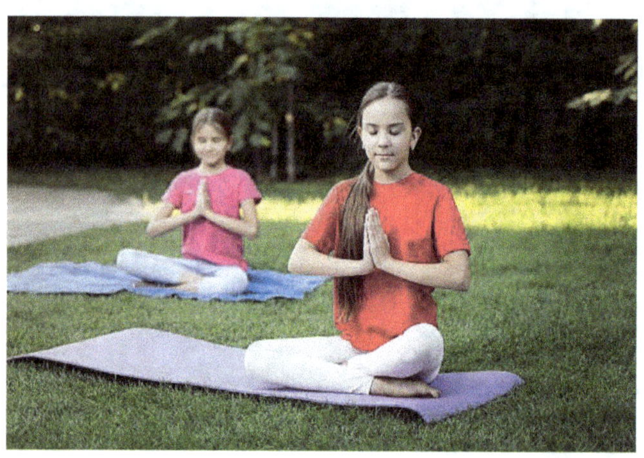

Alternate nostril breathing (Nadi Shodhana):

Technique:

- Sit comfortably with your back straight.
- Use your right thumb to close your right nostril and inhale deeply through your left.
- Close your left nostril with your ring finger, release your right nose, and exhale.
- Continue swapping nostrils for many cycles.

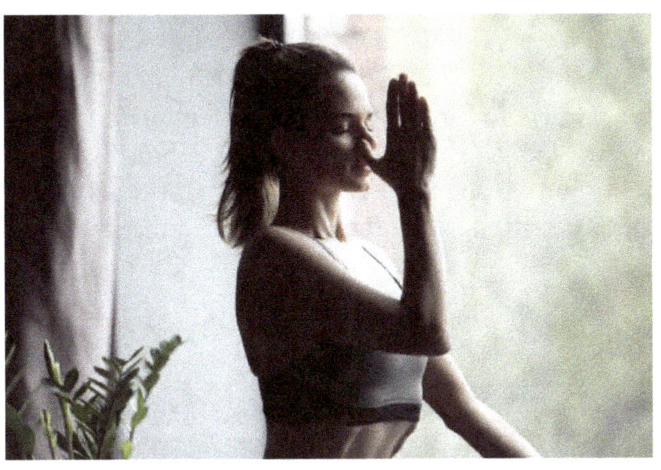

Belly Breathing with Visualization

Technique: Place your hands on your belly and shut your eyes. Inhale deeply through your nose, picturing your breath filling your stomach like a balloon inflating. Exhale gently through your lips while picturing the balloon deflating. Concentrate on the feeling of expanding and releasing with each breath.

2.2 Body Scan and Grounding Exercises.

Body scans and grounding exercises are effective somatic activities for increasing body awareness and promoting stability and presence. This article discusses the intricacies of these activities with eloquent explanations and detailed examples.

Body Scan:

Body scan refers to carefully devoting attention to various sections of the body and examining feelings without judgment or response. This technique promotes awareness and strengthens the link between the mind and body.

Technique:

- Start by choosing a comfortable sitting or sleeping posture.
- Please close your eyes and focus on your breath, allowing it to flow freely.
- Begin at the top of your head and gradually scan downward, noting any feelings or regions of tension.
- Allow relaxation and release with each breath while scanning down to your toes.

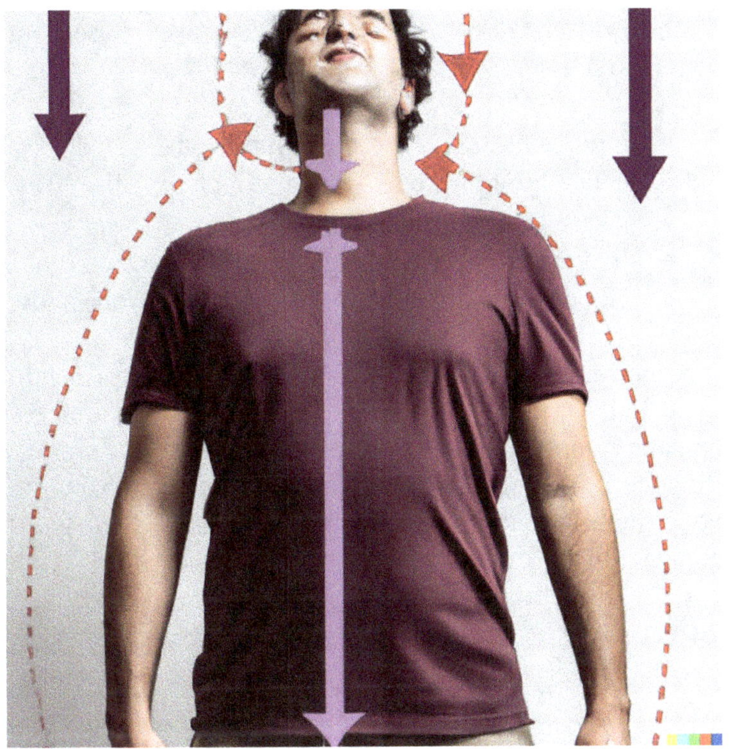

Grounding Exercises:

Grounding exercises help center the mind and body in the present moment, promoting stability and safety. These activities often involve connecting with the earth or using the senses to generate a sense of groundedness.

Technique 1: Rooting to the Earth - Stand tall, feet hip-width apart. Imagine roots growing from the soles of your feet deep into the soil, securely holding you in place. Take deep breaths and feel the soil underneath you.

Technique 2: 5-4-3-2-1 Grounding Exercise - Use your senses to notice:

- You can see five objects around you.
- There are four items you can touch or feel.
- Three things you can hear.
- You can smell two things.
- Concentrate on one flavor or feeling in your body.

Incorporating body scans and grounding exercises into your daily routine will help you develop awareness, presence, and resilience in facing life's adversities. Practice consistently and see the significant impacts on your mind, body, and soul as you strengthen your connection to yourself and the world around you.

2.3 Core Activation and Stability Exercises

Core activation and stability exercises are essential to somatic practices since they strengthen the muscles supporting the spine and pelvis while encouraging balance and alignment. These exercises build physical strength and foster a greater feeling of body awareness and proprioception. Discuss these activities in depth, supported by vivid explanations and detailed examples.

Pelvic Tilt:

Pelvic tilt exercises work the lower back, abdomen, and pelvis muscles to improve spinal stability and alignment.

Technique:

- Lie on your back, legs bent, feet flat on the floor.
- Inhale to prepare, then exhale while softly pressing your lower back into the floor and tilting your pelvis backward.
- Hold for a few seconds, then inhale and return to neutral.

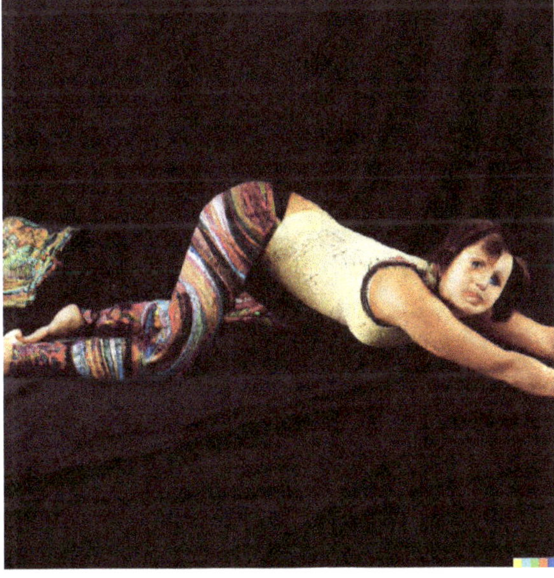

Dead Bug:

Dead bug exercises work the core muscles while demanding stability and coordination, which helps to improve posture and avoid lower back problems.

Technique:

Lie on your back, arms stretched toward the sky, legs lifted, knees bent at 90 degrees. Slowly drop one arm and the opposing leg to the floor, keeping your lower back flat against the ground. Return to the starting position and repeat on the other side.

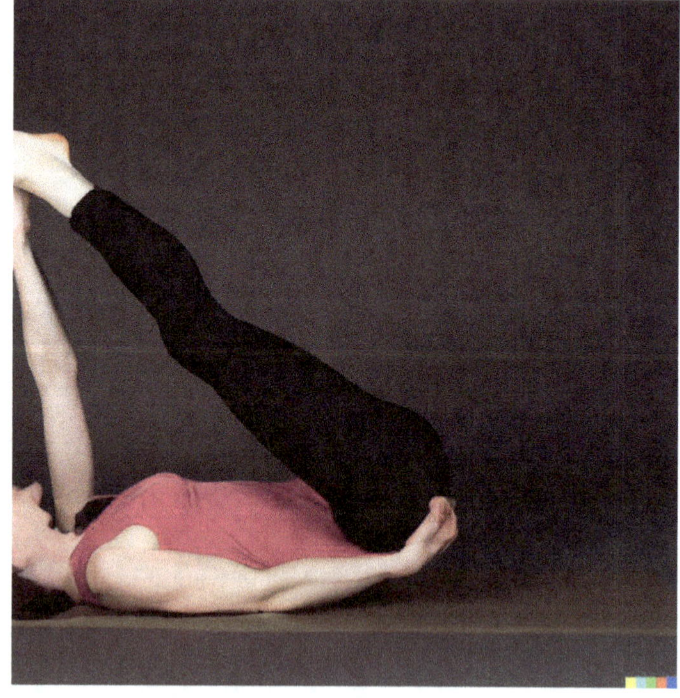

Plank:

The plank is a traditional core stability exercise that works the muscles in the belly, back, shoulders, and glutes, increasing overall strength and stability.

Technique:

Begin in a push-up stance, hands exactly beneath shoulders, and body straight from head to heels. Engage your core muscles and maintain this posture, avoiding drooping or arching.

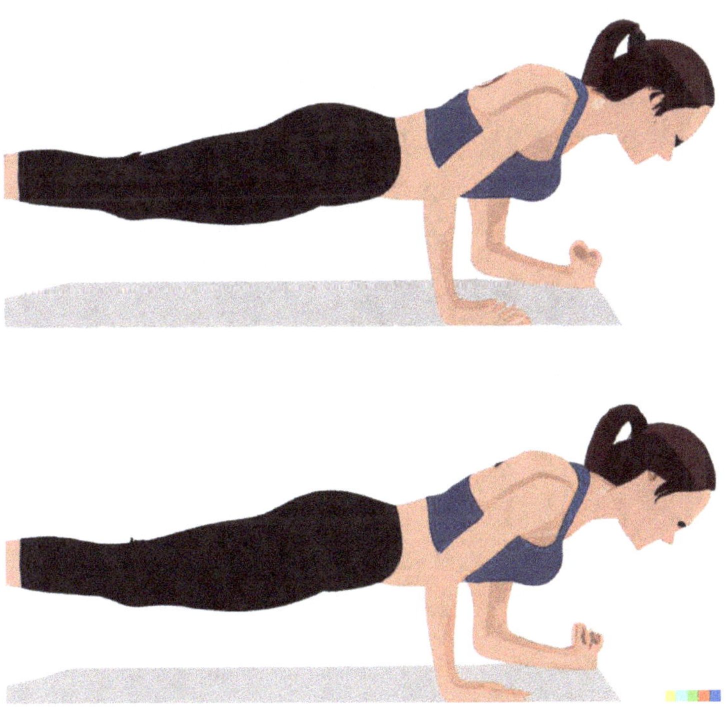

Bird Dogs:

Bird dog movements help to enhance core stability and coordination while also targeting the back and glute muscles.

Technique:

Begin on your hands and knees, placing your wrists under your shoulders and your knees under your hips. Extend one arm forward and the opposing leg backward, keeping your spine neutral. Hold for a few seconds, then return to your starting position and repeat on the other side.

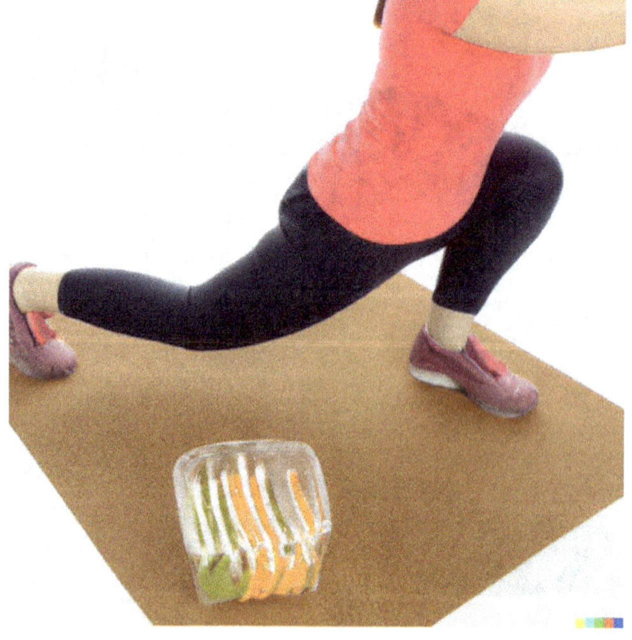

Including these core activation and stability exercises in your regimen may strengthen your foundation, improve your posture, and increase your general body awareness and stability. Practice regularly and see how your physical strength, balance, and alignment improve.

2.4 Motion Exploration for Body Alignment

Movement exploration for body alignment is a dynamic activity that encourages people to experiment with various motions and postures to achieve optimum alignment, flexibility, and coordination. Participants in mindful Movement have a better knowledge of their bodies and become more conscious of their posture and movement patterns. Below, we will go over the specifics of movement exploration, backed by dynamic explanations and detailed examples.

Cat-Cow Stretch:

The cat-cow stretch is a mild yoga-inspired practice that increases spinal mobility and alignment.

Technique:

Begin on your hands and knees, placing your wrists under your shoulders and your knees under your hips. Inhale while arching your back, lowering your belly to the floor, and elevating your eyes (cow position). Exhale while rounding your back, lowering your chin to your chest, and pulling your belly button toward your spine (cat stance). Flow between these two postures, synchronizing your breath and Movement.

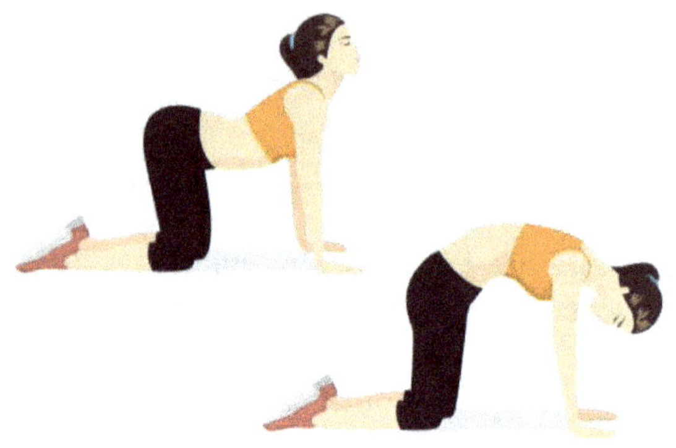

Standing Forward Fold:

The standing forward fold stretches the hamstrings and spine while aligning and extending the back body.

Technique: Stand tall with your feet hip-width apart. Inhale to extend your spine, then exhale as you bend at the hips and fold forward, bringing your hands to the floor or resting them on your shins. Keep your knees slightly bent as required to maintain a neutral spine. Relax your head and neck and let gravity deepen the stretch.

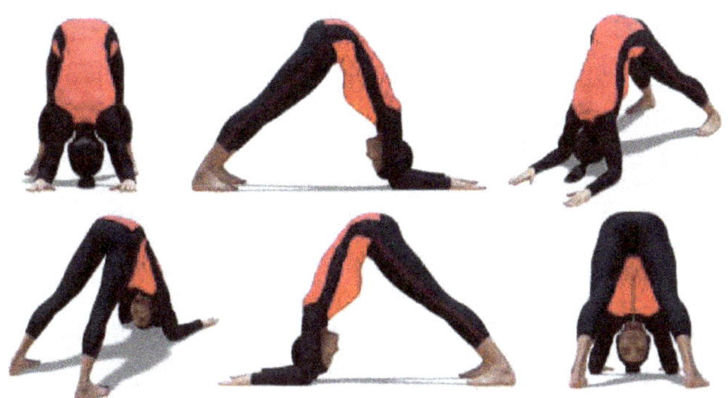

Side Bend Stretch:

Side bend stretches work the muscles on the sides of the body, improving lateral flexibility and alignment.

Technique: Stand tall, feet hip-width apart, arms extended high. Inhale to lengthen your spine, then exhale while leaning to one side, resulting in a nice stretch down the opposing side of your body. Keep both feet planted and your shoulders relaxed. Inhale to return to the center, then repeat on the other side.

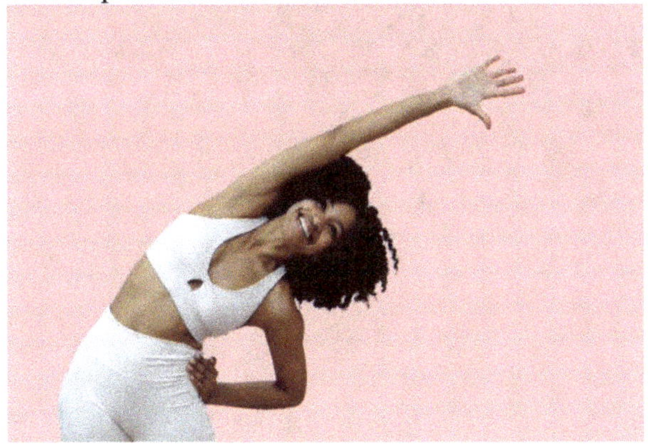

Spinal twist:

Spinal twists increase spinal mobility and alignment while stretching the back and torso muscles.

Technique:

- Sit tall with your legs stretched in front of you.
- Bend one knee and put the foot on the outside of the opposing thigh.
- Inhale to lengthen your spine, then exhale as you twist towards the bent knee, resting your opposite hand on the floor behind you for support.
- Hold the twist for a few breaths before repeating on the other side.

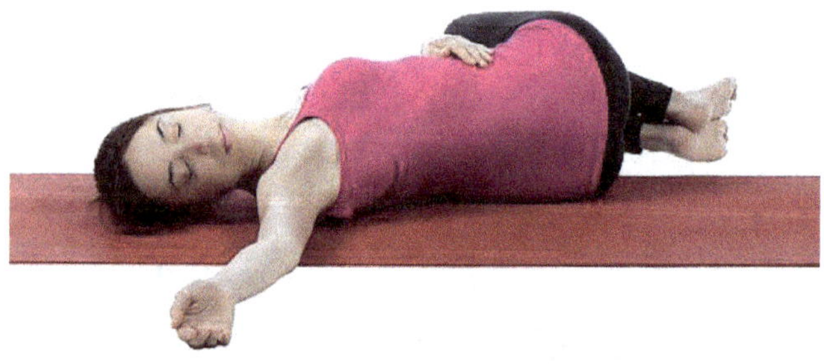

2.5 Promoting Mindfulness in Physical Activity

Mindfulness in physical exercise entails paying close attention to the body's motions, sensations, and surroundings. Individuals who practice mindfulness while exercising may strengthen their connection with their body, improve their performance, and get more happiness and satisfaction from their activities. Let's look at methods to cultivate mindfulness during physical activity:

Cultivate Intention.

Before beginning physical exercise, take a minute to create an aim for your practice. You may wish to attain this particular objective, such as increased flexibility, reduced stress, or a commitment to being present and attentive during your exercise.

Begin with Breath Awareness:

Start your physical exercise by concentrating on your breathing. Consider the pattern of your inhales and exhales as you move, allowing your breath to lead and support you. When your mind wanders, use your breath as an anchor to bring it back to the present.

Tune into Sensations.

Pay special attention to your body's feelings while moving. Consider the sensation of your muscles contracting and relaxing, the rhythm of your pulse, and the input from your joints and limbs. Be curious and nonjudgmental, allowing yourself to completely feel each sensation without attempting to modify or improve anything.

Stay present:

Stay present in each moment of your physical activity rather than getting caught up in ideas about the past or future. Concentrate on the feelings of Movement as they occur in real-time, avoiding distractions or worry. If your thoughts stray, gently bring your focus back to the current moment.

Practice mindful Movement:

Engage in physical exercise with attentive awareness, paying close attention to every Movement and posture. Note your body's alignment, movement quality, and any points of strain or resistance. Allow your actions to flow freely without hurrying or pushing them.

Embrace challenges.

Approach obstacles and difficulties in physical exercise with an open and receptive mindset. Rather than being irritated or disappointed, consider their chances for development and learning. Consider how you react to physical and emotional obstacles and develop resilience and tenacity in adversity.

Appreciate the experience:

Take the time to embrace the experience of physical exercise, recognizing the advantages it provides for your body, mind, and soul. Note any pleasure, success, or satisfaction sensations during and after your exercise. Cultivate thankfulness for your body's capacity to move and the chance to participate in physical activities.

Integrating mindfulness into your physical exercise regimen may improve your general wellbeing and strengthen your connection with your body. Practice these strategies daily to enhance your attention during workouts and feel the transformational power of mindful Movement.

Chapter 3: Targeted Somatic Exercises for Weight Loss

3.1 Dynamic Movement Sequences for Strength and Flexibility.

Dynamic movement sequences are fluid motions that mix strength-building workouts with stretches to improve flexibility. These sequences increase athletic performance and encourage mindfulness, coordination, and body awareness. Let's look in depth at how to do dynamic movement sequences for strength and flexibility, complete with vibrant explanations and detailed examples.

Sun Salutations (Surya Namaskar):

Sun Salutation is a traditional yoga sequence that moves dynamically through several positions to improve strength, flexibility, and balance.

Technique:

- Start in Mountain Pose (Tadasana) with your feet together and your arms by your sides.

- Inhale and raise your arms upwards, arching back slightly into a moderate backbend (Upward Salute).
- Exhale and fold forward into a Forward Fold (Uttanasana). Inhale to rise halfway and stretch the spine (Half Forward Fold),
- then exhale to place your hands and return to Plank Pose. Lower into Chaturanga and inhale to rise into Upward-Facing Dog (Urdhva Mukha Svanasana).
- Exhale and elevate your hips into a Downward-Facing Dog (Adho Mukha Svanasana).
- Repeat the routine, transitioning effortlessly from one stance to the next.

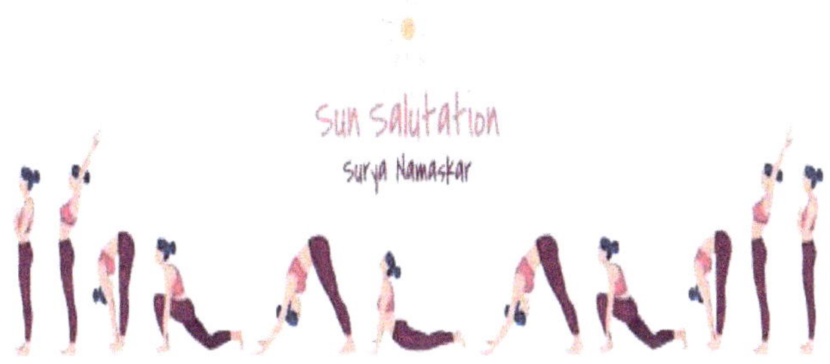

Dynamic Warrior Flow:

Warrior Flow is a dynamic practice that blends warrior postures with flowing movements to strengthen and stretch the lower body.

Begin in Warrior II (Virabhadrasana II) with the right leg forward, the left leg behind, and arms parallel to the floor. Inhale as you straighten your right leg and raise your arms above, rising through your chest (reverse warrior). Exhale as you bend your right knee and sweep your arms down and forward to enter Warrior I (Virabhadrasana I). Inhale to return to Warrior II, and exhale to resume Downward-Facing Dog. Repeat on the other side.

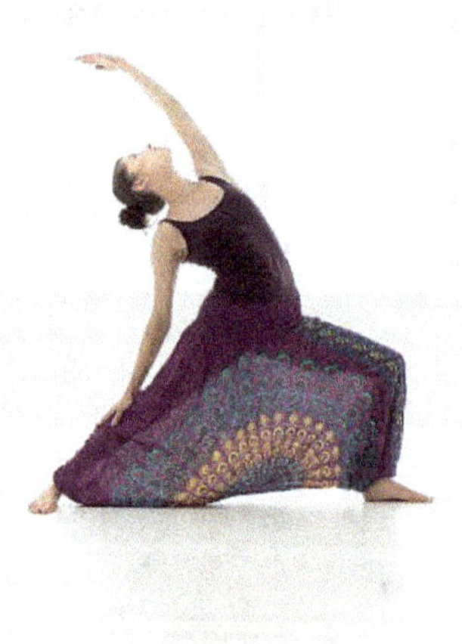

Dynamic Lunge Sequence:

The Dynamic Lunge Sequence improves lower-body strength and flexibility by combining lunging motions with dynamic stretches.
Starting in a standing posture, step back into a deep lunge while lowering your right knee to the floor. Inhale to raise

your arms upwards, reaching for the heavens. Exhale as you rotate your body to the left, placing your right elbow on the outside of your left knee. Inhale to return to the center, then exhale to take a step forward. Repeat on the opposite side.

Dynamic Bridge Flow:

The Dynamic Bridge Flow routine works the back, glutes, and hamstrings while increasing spinal mobility and flexibility.

Technique: Begin by reclining on your back, knees bent, and feet hip-width apart. Inhale as you elevate your hips to the sky, entering Bridge Pose (Setu Bandhasana). Exhale as you drop your hips back to the ground. Inhale and raise your hips again, raising your arms aloft and stretching your fingers. Exhale to bring your hips and arms back down. Repeat the pattern, moving gently with your breath.

Including these dynamic movement sequences in your exercise program may improve your strength and flexibility while developing mindfulness and body awareness. Practice these sequences regularly to experience the transforming effects of dynamic Movement on both your body and mind.

3.2 Spinal Mobility and Alignment Techniques

Spinal mobility and alignment practices are critical for keeping your spine healthy, increasing flexibility, and avoiding injuries. These treatments aim to move the vertebrae of the spine, correct imbalances, and encourage ideal alignment for general health. Discuss these strategies in depth, backed with vibrant explanations and detailed examples.

Seated Spinal Twist:

Seated spinal twists are an efficient way to improve mobility in the thoracic and lumbar spines while extending the muscles along the back and sides of the body.

Technique: Begin by sitting with your legs out in front of you. Bend your right knee and cross it over the left leg, with the foot flat on the ground outside the left thigh. Inhale to stretch the spine, then exhale as you twist to the right, with your left elbow on the outside of the right knee and your right hand on the floor behind you for support. Hold the twist for several breaths before switching sides.

Benefits: Seated spinal twists relieve back muscular tension, increase spinal mobility, and promote digestion and detoxification.

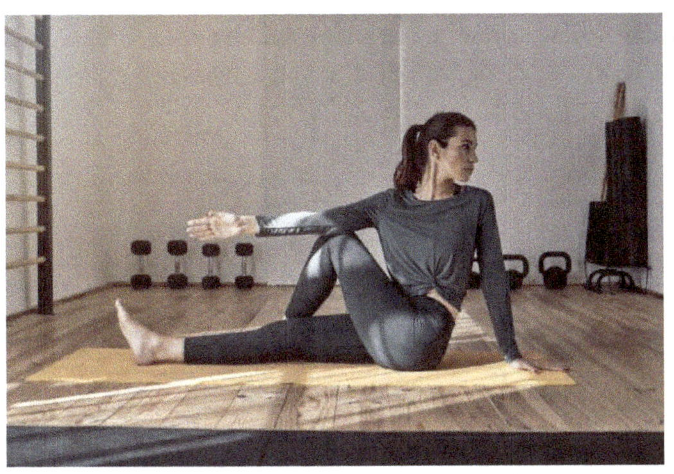

Cobra pose (bhujangasana):

Cobra posture is a backbend that works the spine, belly, and chest muscles, increasing flexibility and mobility in the thoracic and lumbar areas.

Technique:

- Face down on the mat, hands under shoulders, elbows close to the torso.
- Inhale as you squeeze your hands together to elevate your chest off the floor, keeping your elbows slightly bent and your shoulders relaxed.
- Draw the shoulder blades together and lift through the sternum to extend the spine.
- Hold for a few breaths before exhaling and lowering back down.

Benefits: The cobra position stretches the front body muscles while strengthening the back, improving posture, and reducing spinal stress.

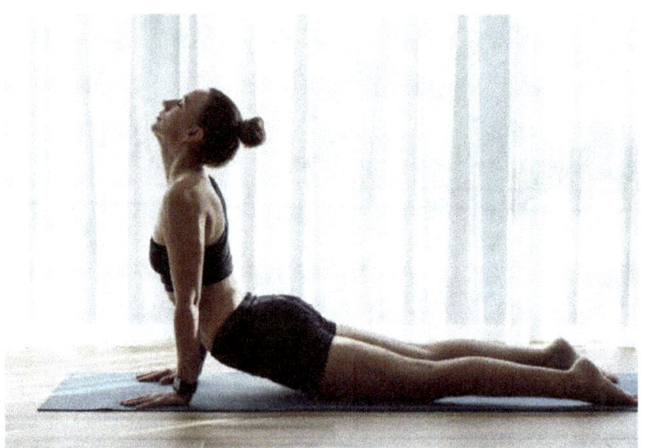

Thread the Needle Pose (Parsva Balasana).

Thread the needle position is a gentle twist that works the spine, shoulders, and neck muscles, increasing mobility and relieving tension in the upper back.

Begin on your hands and knees, placing your wrists under your shoulders and your knees under your hips. Inhale to raise your right arm to the ceiling, then exhale to thread it beneath the left arm, dropping the right shoulder and ear to the mat. Hold the stretch for a few breaths, pushing your left hand firmly into the floor for support. Inhale to return to the beginning position, then repeat on the other side.

Benefits: Thread the needle position reduces upper back and shoulder tension, improves spinal mobility, and reduces stress and anxiety.

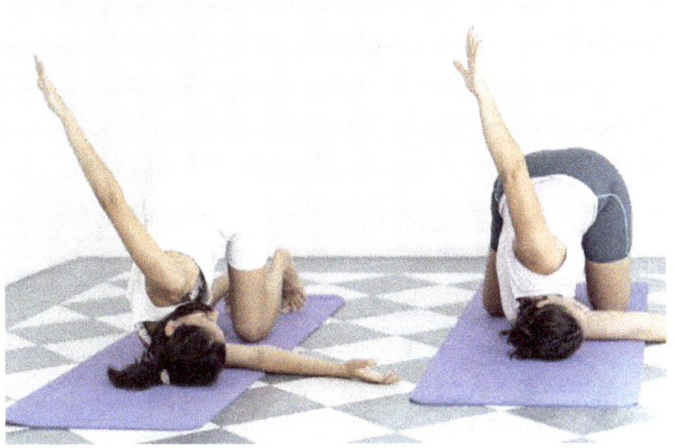

Supported bridge pose (Setu Bandhasana):

Supported Bridge Pose is a moderate backbend that extends the spine, expands the chest, and relieves lower back and hip tension.

Technique:

- Lie on your back, knees bent and feet hip-width apart, arms at your sides.
- Inhale while pressing your feet into the ground and lifting your hips to the sky, using a yoga block or bolster to support your sacrum.
- Maintain knee alignment over ankles while using the glutes and abdominal muscles.

- Hold the position for a few breaths before exhaling and lowering the hips back down.

Benefits: Supported bridge posture improves spinal flexibility, reduces lower back discomfort, and promotes relaxation and stress reduction.

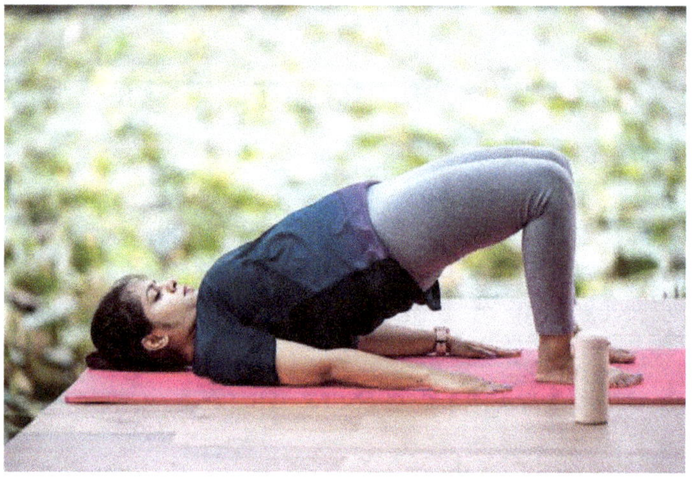

Incorporating these extra spinal mobility and alignment practices into your routine can improve flexibility, mobility, and general spinal health. Practice these daily to get the full spectrum of health and wellness advantages.

3.4 Mindful Eating Strategies and Somatic Awareness

Mindful eating entails establishing a thorough awareness of the current food experience. In contrast, somatic awareness entails tuning into the body's feelings and messages. Combining these two activities may result in a deeper connection with food and a better understanding of our bodies' needs and reactions. Let's go over these principles in depth, highlighting their significance and how they may be incorporated into everyday life:

Mindfulness Eating Practices:

Engage All Senses: Mindful eating starts before food enters the mouth. Take a minute to study the food's sight, fragrance, and texture. Observe any feelings of hunger or anticipation that occur.

Slow Down:

Eat carefully and relish every mouthful.
- Note the tastes, textures, and feelings as you chew.
- Take intervals between bites to listen to your body and analyze your appetite and fullness.
- Listen to your body's hunger and satiety signals. Eat when you're hungry, and stop when you're full, even if there's still food on your plate. Learn the difference between bodily hunger and emotional or environmental urges to eat.

- Be present: Avoid distractions when eating. Turn off the displays, put away technological gadgets, and concentrate entirely on the process of eating. Eating attentively helps you to appreciate the nutrients and pleasure that food brings completely.

Practice Gratitude: Take a minute to be grateful for the meal you will consume. Cultivating gratitude for the sustenance and energy it provides may improve the eating experience and foster a good attitude toward food.

Somatic awareness:

Body feelings: Somatic awareness is awareness of one's emotions and impulses. Pay attention to your body's sensations before, during, and after eating. Take note of bodily feelings like hunger, fullness, contentment, or pain.

Emotional Awareness:

Be mindful of any feelings or ideas when eating. Determine if you're eating out of habit, boredom, stress, or other emotional causes. Mindful eating entails recognizing these feelings without judgment and deciding how to react.

Somatic awareness promotes intuitive eating by allowing you to listen to your body's natural cues and signals. Learn to trust your body's wisdom and make eating choices that meet your physical and emotional requirements.

Body Feedback:

Notice how various meals make you feel. Consider how certain meals stimulate you while others make you feel sluggish or unpleasant. Use this input to decide what and how much to consume.

Nonjudgmental Observation:

Approach bodily awareness with curiosity and without judgment. Observe your body's feelings and reactions without classifying them as positive or negative. This open-mindedness enables you to learn from each event and make changes as necessary.

By combining mindful eating techniques and somatic awareness into your daily routine, you may develop a stronger connection with your body and food, resulting in better physical and mental health. Practice these practices daily to establish a more harmonious connection with food and a higher feeling of vigor and balance.

3.5 Stress and Relaxation Techniques for Weight Management

Stress reduction and relaxation strategies are important in weight control because they assist in minimizing stress-induced eating, developing mindful eating habits, and improving general wellbeing. When stressed, our bodies produce cortisol, which causes increased appetite, desires for unhealthy foods, and weight gain. Implementing stress reduction and relaxation strategies into your daily routine may improve your stress management and support your weight control objectives. Let's look at these strategies in depth, with explicit explanations and examples:

Deep breathing exercises:

Deep breathing techniques, such as diaphragmatic or belly breathing, trigger the body's relaxation response, reducing tension and promoting calm.

Find a quiet, comfortable place to sit or lie down. Close your eyes and lay one hand on your stomach, the other on your chest. Inhale deeply through your nose, letting your stomach expand as you fill your lungs with air. Exhale slowly through your lips, allowing your tummy to compress softly. Repeat this deep breathing pattern for a few minutes, concentrating on the rhythm of your breath and releasing tension with each exhale.

Progressive Muscle Relaxation:

PMR is a method of systematically tensing and releasing various muscle groups to promote physical and mental calm.

Example:

- Begin by sitting or lying down in a comfortable posture.

- Begin with your feet. Progressively tighten the muscles in your toes, holding for a few seconds before releasing and relaxing.
- Ascend, tense, and release each muscle group, including the calves, thighs, belly, chest, arms, shoulders, neck, and face.
- Pay attention to the feelings of tension melting away as you relax each muscle area, which promotes general relaxation and stress reduction.

Mindful Meditation:

Mindfulness meditation entails paying close attention to the current moment while fostering awareness of thoughts, emotions, and body sensations without judgment.

Find a quiet area and sit comfortably with your eyes closed. Focus on your breathing, feeling the sensations of each inhale and exhale. When your mind wanders (as it will certainly do), gently redirect Your concentration to your breath without judgment. Practice being present in each moment, noting and releasing ideas and feelings as they emerge. Regular mindfulness meditation may help decrease stress, develop self-awareness, and promote emotional balance, which benefits healthy weight control.

Guided imagery and visualization:

Guided imagery is a relaxing technique and reduces stress by mentally envisioning serene, tranquil sights or events.

Close your eyes and envision yourself in a peaceful environment like a beach, forest, or hilltop. Imagine yourself surrounded by beauty and peace, absorbing the sights, sounds, and fragrances of your imagined surroundings. Allow yourself to get immersed in the experience, observing how it feels to be utterly calm and at ease. Guided imagery may help you divert your attention away from stresses and produce a feeling of calm and wellbeing, which can help you maintain good eating habits and achieve your weight loss objectives.

Yoga & Tai Chi:

Yoga and Tai Chi are mind-body activities that use physical Movement and breath awareness to promote relaxation, flexibility, and stress reduction.

Try a mild yoga flow or Tai Chi practice that stresses slow, deliberate movements and careful breathing. Concentrate on the sensations of each Movement as you transition from one posture to the next, allowing tension to dissolve and the mind to calm. These techniques may help lower stress hormones, promote feelings of relaxation, and improve general physical and mental health, all of which contribute to successful weight control.

Adopting these stress-reduction and relaxation strategies into your daily routine may improve stress management, enhance mindfulness, and support good eating habits and weight control objectives. Experiment with various techniques to see what works best for you, and prioritize self-care for maximum health and wellbeing.

Chapter Four: Advanced Somatic Exercise Strategies.

4.1 Progressive Muscle Relaxation to Enhance Body Awareness

Progressive Muscle Relaxation (PMR) is a relaxation method that gradually tenses and releases various muscle groups to induce physical and mental calm. Individuals who practice PMR might gain greater body awareness, detecting stress regions and learning to release it intentionally. Let's go over how to execute PMR in-depth, with expressive explanations and detailed examples:

Preparation:

- Find a quiet, comfortable area to lie down or sit relaxed. Remove all distractions and ensure that you will not be disturbed while practicing.
- Close your eyes and take a few deep breaths to focus yourself before beginning the relaxation practice. Allow your body to relax and release whatever stress you may be harboring.

Starting Position:

- Begin by concentrating on your feet. Take a deep breath and curl your toes firmly, keeping the position for a few seconds. Then, exhale and release the tension, allowing your toes to relax fully.

- Consider the contrast between the sensations of tension and relaxation in your toes. As you release the tension, pay attention to any feelings that arise, such as warmth or tingling.

Progressive muscle tension and relaxation:

- Continue upward to the next muscle group, which may be your calf muscles. Inhale deeply and contract your calves' muscles by pointing your toes upward briefly. Then, exhale and release the tension, allowing your calf muscles to relax fully.
- Again, notice the difference between tension and relaxation in your calves. Consider how the muscles feel when they are tight vs relaxed.

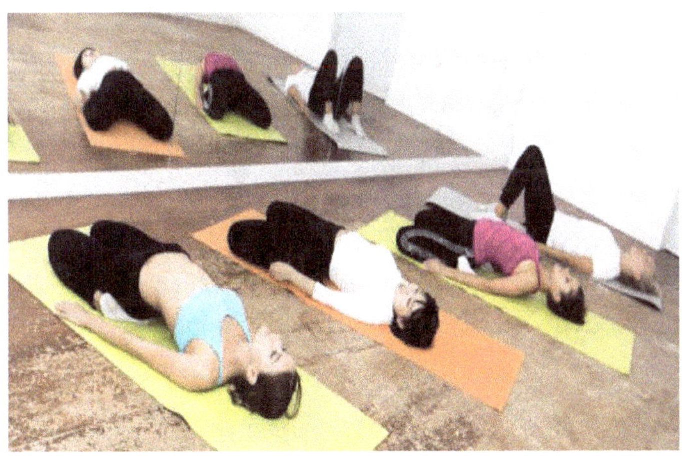

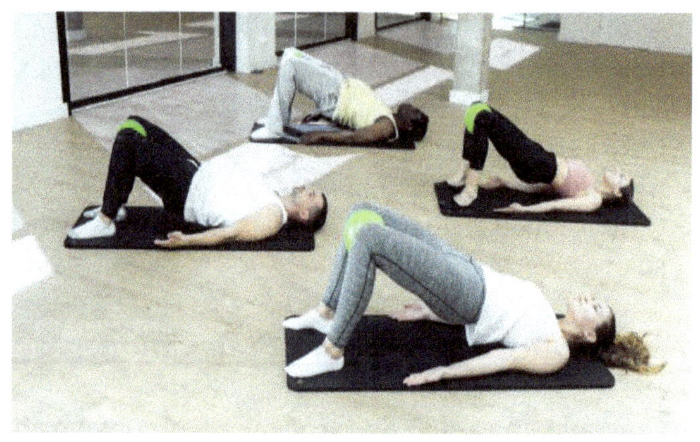

Continuing Through the Body:

- Repeat this method for each major muscle group in the body, such as the thighs, buttocks, belly, chest, back, shoulders, arms, hands, neck, and face.

- As you work through each muscle group, take time to completely contract and release the muscles, paying particular attention to the feelings and distinctions between tension and relaxation.

- Visualize the tension melting away from each muscle area as you release it, enabling your whole body to relax deeper with each repetition.

Closing and Integration:

- After you've finished the progressive relaxation cycle for all muscle groups, spend a few seconds to absorb the general sensation of relaxation and calm in your body.

- Take note of differences in how your body feels now from when you first began the practice. You may feel lighter, more grounded, and more in tune with your body's natural relaxation response.

- When you're ready, gradually return your consciousness to the current moment. Wiggle your fingers and toes, softly extend your limbs, and open your eyes.

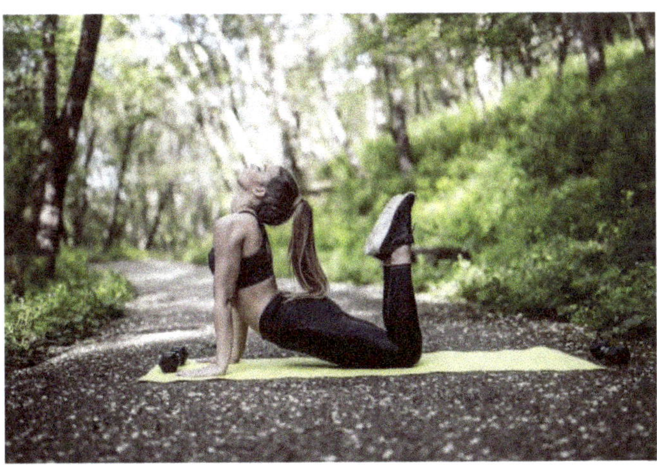

Individuals who practice Progressive Muscle Relaxation (PMR) daily may better understand their bodies, recognize regions of tension, and learn to release tension deliberately. This practice may help manage stress, promote relaxation, and improve general wellbeing. Experiment with PMR and include it in your self-care regimen to experience its transforming effects on both body and mind.

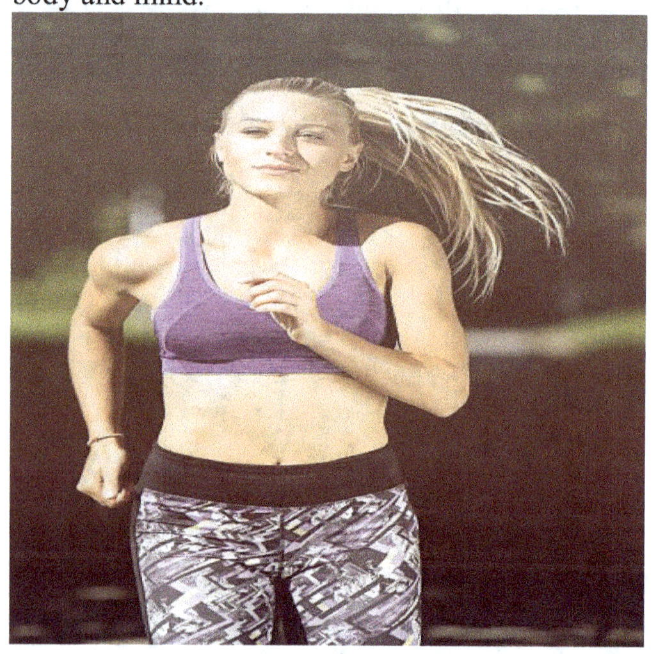

4.2 Functional Movement Patterns for Daily Activities

Functional movement patterns are required for daily tasks with ease, efficiency, and a low risk of harm. These motions combine numerous joints and muscle groups to simulate real-life actions, including walking, squatting, lifting, and reaching. Adding functional movement patterns into your training program may increase your strength, agility, and stability, making everyday tasks easier and more pleasant. Let us investigate available movement patterns in depth, using expressive explanations and examples:

Squatting:

Squatting is a basic movement pattern that includes bending the knees and hips while maintaining the spine straight, similar to sitting down and standing up.

Stand with your feet hip-width apart and toes pointing slightly outward. Bend your knees and hips to lower your body while maintaining your chest raised and your weight in your heels. Lower until your thighs are parallel to the ground or as far as you can comfortably go, then push through your heels to stand back up. Squatting strengthens the lower body muscles, such as the quadriceps, hamstrings, glutes, and calves, which are necessary for sitting, standing, and lifting.

Pushing:

Pushing is pushing an item away from the body by extending the arms and working the muscles in the chest, shoulders, and triceps.

Example: Begin a push-up in a plank stance with hands shoulder-width apart and wrists squarely beneath shoulders. Lower your body to the ground by bending your elbows and keeping them close to your torso. Push yourself back up to the starting posture, arms fully extended. Pushing actions are necessary to open doors, make a shopping cart, and move goods above.
Pulling:

Pulling is pulling an item closer to the body by flexing the arms and engaging the back, shoulders, and biceps muscles.

Perform a bent-over row by standing with your feet hip-width apart and gripping a dumbbell in each hand, palms facing the body. Hinge forward at the hips with your back flat and chest elevated. Bend your elbows and squeeze your shoulder blades together to bring the dumbbells closer to your chest. Lower the weights back down with control. Opening drawers, moving groceries, and closing doors all require pulling actions.

Lunging:

Lunging is a movement in which you stride forward or backward with one leg while erecting your torso, using muscles in your legs, hips, and core.

For example, stand tall with your feet hip-width apart to make a forward lunge. Step forward with one foot, lowering your body by bending both knees so the front thigh is parallel to the ground and the rear knee is just above the floor. Push through the front heel to return to the beginning position, then repeat on the other side. Lunging motions are required for ascending stairs, walking uphill, and bending down to pick up items.
Rotation:

Rotation includes turning the body from side to side, which activates muscles in the core, back, and obliques.
For example, to do a standing torso twist, stand with your feet hip-width apart and arms outstretched in front of you. Rotate your torso to one side, maintaining the hips front and the spine upright. Return to the center, then rotate to the other side. Rotation motions are required for reaching across your body, swinging a golf club, and turning to see behind you while driving.

Adding functional movement patterns to your training program may increase strength, mobility, and stability, simplify daily tasks, and lower your risk of injury. Practice these motions regularly to improve your total functional fitness and experience increased comfort and efficiency in everyday life.

4.3 Integrating Somatics with Cardiovascular Exercise

Integrating somatics into cardiovascular exercise may increase workout efficacy while developing body awareness, mindfulness, and relaxation. Somatics focuses on developing the mind-body connection, reducing tension, and growing movement efficiency, all of which may supplement cardiovascular exercise. Let's take a detailed look at how to include somatics into cardiovascular training, complete with vibrant explanations and illustrations:

Body Scan Warm-up:

Description: Start your cardiovascular exercise with a body scan to become aware of your body's feelings and regions of stress. This allows you to become more conscious of your posture, alignment, and movement patterns before participating in more strenuous activity.

Example: To center yourself, stand straight with your feet hip-width apart, shut your eyes, and take a few deep breaths. Begin with your feet and gradually scan your body from head to toe, noting any areas of stiffness or pain. Before beginning your aerobic activity, use moderate motions to relieve tension and encourage relaxation, such as rolling your shoulders or circling your wrists.

Mindful Walking or Running:

Practice mindful walking or jogging to pay attention to your body's motions and feelings while participating in cardiovascular activity. This allows you to be present in the moment while maintaining perfect form and alignment.

Example: While walking or jogging, concentrate on the feeling of your feet touching the ground, the rhythm of your breath, and the Movement of your arms. Take note of how your body reacts to each step or stride, and change your posture to stay aligned. To improve movement efficiency and lessen the chance of injury, use bodily signals such as relaxing your shoulders or activating your core muscles.

Breathwork Integration:

Incorporate breathing methods into your aerobic activity to improve relaxation, endurance, and concentration. Paying attention to your breath might help you control your heart rate and energy levels when exercising.

To practice deep belly breathing while walking, running, or cycling, inhale deeply with the nose, allowing the belly to expand, and exhale slowly through the mouth, pulling the belly button towards the spine. Synchronize your breath with exercise to establish a consistent rhythm to help your cardiovascular efforts. Use breath awareness to be present and relaxed, particularly during difficult periods or uphill climbs.

Dynamic stretch and mobility drills:

Description: Incorporate dynamic stretching and mobility routines into your cardiovascular warm-up to prepare your muscles and joints for action while increasing flexibility and range of motion.

For example, before beginning your aerobic activity, do dynamic motions like leg swings, arm circles, or hip rotations. Concentrate on gentle, controlled motions that gently mobilize the joints and muscles without pushing or straining. Use somatic cues to listen to your body's input and change your actions appropriately to avoid injury and improve performance.

Cooldown and Body Awareness Reflection:

Description: After cardiovascular activity, cool down to gradually drop your heart rate and encourage relaxation. Take this opportunity to reflect on your body's experiences and any insights acquired from the exercise.

For example, after your aerobic workout, slowly transition to a gentle stroll or jog to let your body return to rest gradually. Use this time to check in with your body and observe any changes in muscular tension, breathing patterns, or energy levels. Reflect on your experience, recognizing any movement quality changes or awareness resulting from somatic integration.

Illustrations: [Images of people participating in cardiovascular exercise using somatic signals and practices, including mindful walking, deep breathing, dynamic stretching, and contemplation of body awareness. Arrows and comments draw attention to important areas of emphasis, such as posture, alignment, and movement efficiency.

Incorporating somatics into your cardiovascular workout program may strengthen the mind-body connection, increase movement quality, and promote relaxation and wellbeing. Experiment with these approaches to see how they improve your entire training experience and help you meet your health and fitness objectives.

4.4 Tailoring Somatic Exercise Routines to Individual Needs

Personalizing somatic exercise regimens is critical for meeting individual requirements, objectives, and limits. Bodily exercises concentrate on increasing body awareness, relieving tension, and refining movement patterns, making them adaptable to various talents and preferences. Individuals who adjust somatic exercise regimens to their requirements might find higher efficacy, pleasure, and long-term success in their fitness journey. Let's go over how to tailor somatic workout regimens in detail:

Assessment and goal-setting:

Assessment: Begin by determining the individual's current fitness level, movement patterns, areas of tension or pain, and particular goals.

Goal Setting: Work with the person to develop specific, attainable objectives consistent with their interests, preferences, and ambitions. Goals may include increasing flexibility, lowering stress, improving posture, relieving chronic pain, or improving general health.

Customized Exercise Selection:

Exercise Selection: Choose somatic exercises that cater to the individual's specific requirements, interests, and objectives. Choose workouts that address particular muscle groups, movement patterns, or stress points indicated during the evaluation.

Range and Progress: Use a range of bodily exercises to keep the regimen interesting and effective. As the individual's fitness levels improve, the intensity, length, or complexity of the workouts gradually increase.

Adaptations and modifications:

Adaptations: Change the somatic exercises to meet any physical limits, injuries, or medical issues that the person may have. Provide alternate motions or modifications that lessen pain while delivering the intended results.
Equipment & Props: Use yoga blocks, straps, or foam rollers to maintain good posture, provide stability, or deepen stretches.

Mindful Cueing and Feedback:

Thoughtful Cueing: Use clear, brilliant cues to help the person through each somatic exercise, focusing on good alignment, breath awareness, and mindful Movement.

Comments: Provide constructive comments and encouragement to assist the person in refining their technique, increasing their body awareness, and maximizing the efficacy of each exercise.

Individualized Progress Plan:

Progression Plan: Create a tailored progression plan that details how the individual will proceed through their somatic exercise program over time. Set precise goals, benchmarks, or checkpoints to monitor progress and change the routine as necessary.

Periodic Evaluation: Conduct regular assessments to examine the individual's requirements, objectives, and progress. Modify the somatic exercise regimen as needed to guarantee ongoing challenge, progress, and alignment with the individual's changing needs and goals.

Encouragement and empowerment:

Encouragement: Provide constant encouragement, support, and inspiration to help clients stick to their somatic exercise practice. Celebrate every accomplishment, no matter how minor, and recognize the individual's efforts and devotion.

Empowerment: Provide the person with information, resources, and tools to help them take control of their fitness journey and achieve long-term success. Encourage self-reflection, mindfulness, and self-care techniques to improve general wellbeing outside the exercise regimen.

Appendix:

A.1 Example Somatic Exercise Routines

Here are some example somatic exercise regimens that anyone may add to their daily or weekly routine:

Morning Wake-Up Routine:

Goal: To energize the body and mind, relieve stress, and increase mobility.

Exercises:

Standing Forward Fold:

- Stand with your feet hip-width apart, bend at the hips, and fold forward, allowing the upper body to hang freely.
- Allow your arms to dangle or grab opposite elbows.
- Take deep breaths and sway from side to side.

Cat-Cow Stretch:

- Assume a tabletop posture on hands and knees. Inhale, arch your back and elevate your chest and tailbone toward the ceiling (cow posture). Exhale, round the back, and tuck the chin into the chest (cat stance). Repeat for a few breaths.

Seated Spinal Twist:

- Sit cross-legged on the floor. Inhale to stretch the spine, then exhale to twist to one side, with one hand behind and the other on the opposing knee. Hold for a few breaths, and then swap sides.

Neck Rolls:

- Sit or stand comfortably and gently lower the chin to the chest.
- Roll your head gently from side to side, stopping at any tight regions.
- Repeat in the other way.

Midday Mobility Break:

Goal: Reduce stiffness from extended sitting, improve circulation, and clear the mind.

Exercises:

Seated Shoulder Rolls:

- Sit upright on a chair, feet flat on the floor.
- Roll your shoulders forward, up, back, and down in a smooth circular motion.

- Repeat numerous times, then reverse direction.

Hip Circles:

- Stand with feet hip-width apart and hands on hips.
- Circle the hips clockwise and then reverse.
- Concentrate on maintaining the Movement smooth and controlled.

Side Bend Stretch:

- Stand with your feet hip-width apart and arms stretched above.
- Lean gently to one side, feeling a stretch down the side of your body.
- Hold for a few breaths, and then swap sides.

Wrist Flexor Stretch:

- Extend one arm before you, palm facing down. With the other hand, gently push the fingers on the body until a stretch is felt in the forearm. Hold for a few breaths, and then swap arms.

Evening Relaxation Routine:

The goal is to release accumulated stress from the day, encourage relaxation, and prepare for a good night's sleep.

Exercises:

Child's Pose:

- Begin by knees, then sit back on the heels and fold the upper body forward, stretching the arms out in front or beside the torso. Hold for a few breaths, concentrating on deep abdominal breathing.

Legs-up-the-Wall Pose:

- Sit with one side of your body against a wall.
- Swing the legs up the wall while lying on your back, creating an L-shape with your body.
- Relax the arms at your sides and shut your eyes.
- Hold for 5-10 minutes, taking calm, even breaths.

Savasana (Corpse Pose):

- Lie flat on your back, legs outstretched, arms at your sides, palms up.
- Close your eyes and allow your body to relax, fully releasing tension from head to toe.
- Hold this stance for 5-10 minutes, concentrating on deep relaxation.

Deep Breathing:

- Sit or sleep comfortably, with one hand on the abdomen and the other on the chest. Inhale deeply through the nose, extending the abdomen first, then the chest. Exhale gently through your lips, allowing the stomach to decompress. Repeat for many minutes, concentrating on the rhythm of your breath.

These example somatic exercise routines may be tailored to individual tastes, skills, and time limits. Encourage people to listen to their bodies and change activities to meet their requirements. Somatic activities help you become more aware of your body, decrease stress, and enhance your general wellbeing.

A.2 Glossary of Somatic and Weight Loss Terms

Somatics is the study of the body as seen from the inside, emphasizing the interior experience of Movement, sensation, and posture.

Body Awareness is the capacity to sense and comprehend the sensations, emotions, and locations of one's body in space.

Mind-Body Connection: This term refers to the interaction between mind and body and focuses on how thoughts, emotions, and beliefs affect physical health and wellbeing.

Weight Loss is the decrease of body weight, usually accomplished through a combination of food changes, exercise, and lifestyle adjustments.

Body Positivity is a movement that promotes acceptance and respect for all body shapes, questions traditional beauty standards, and encourages self-love and acceptance.

Self-compassion is treating oneself with care, understanding, and acceptance, particularly during adversity or failure.

Progressive Muscle Relaxation is a relaxation method in which various muscle groups are tensed and subsequently relaxed to induce physical and mental calm.

Core Activation: Engaging the core muscles, which include the abdominals, obliques, and lower back, helps stabilize the spine and facilitate Movement.

Functional Movement is exercises that simulate normal motions and activities to enhance strength, balance, flexibility, and coordination for everyday use.

Cardiovascular Exercise: Physical activities that raise the heart rate and respiratory rate, such as walking, jogging, cycling, or swimming, to develop cardiovascular fitness and endurance.

Flexibility is the capacity of a joint or set of joints to move through a complete range of motion, which may be enhanced by stretching and mobility exercises.

Strength Training: Exercises that enhance muscular strength, power, and endurance, usually including resistance training with weights, resistance bands, or bodyweight exercises.

Body composition refers to the percentage of fat, muscle, bone, and other tissues in the body and is often used to assess general health and fitness.

Metabolism is the process by which the body turns food and nutrients into energy, which affects weight control and general health.

Nutrition studies how food and nutrients influence the body's growth, development, and health, including dietary choices and behaviors that promote maximum wellbeing.

Portion control regulates food portion sizes to reduce calorie intake and facilitate weight management.

Mindful eating involves paying attention to the sensory experience of eating, such as taste, texture, and hunger signals, to encourage healthy eating habits and weight control.

Stress control: Techniques and techniques for reducing and dealing with stress may affect eating habits and weight control.

Restorative practices are activities or exercises that encourage relaxation, stress reduction, and healing, such as meditation, deep breathing, or gentle stretching.

Self-care refers to practices and activities emphasizing physical, emotional, and mental wellbeing, such as exercise, relaxation, and activities that offer pleasure and satisfaction.

Two weeks Somatic Exercise planner

Week 1:

Day 1:

Morning: Gentle Stretching Routine (10 minutes).
Afternoon: Core Activation and Stability Exercises (15 min)
Evening: Relaxation Techniques for Stress Reduction (10 min)

Day 2:

Morning: Dynamic Movement Sequences for Strength and Flexibility (20 min)
Afternoon: Mindful Eating and Somatic Awareness (15 minutes)
Evening: Progressive Muscle Relaxation for Deeper Body Awareness (10 min)

Day 3:

Morning: Breathing Techniques for Somatic Awareness (10 min)
Afternoon: Body Scan and Grounding Exercises (15 min)
Evening: Spinal Mobility and Alignment Techniques (10 Minutes)

Day 4:

Morning: Functional Movement Patterns for Everyday Activities (20 min)
Afternoon: Integrating Somatics into Cardiovascular Exercise (15 min)
Evening: Mindfulness and Physical Activity (10 minutes)

Day 5:

Morning: Pelvic Floor Engagement and Core Strengthening Exercises (15 Minutes)
Afternoon: Movement Exploration for Body Alignment (20 min)
Evening: Stress Reduction and Relaxation Techniques (10 Minutes)

Weekend:

Day 6: Restorative Practices and Self-Care (gentle yoga or a nature walk).
Day 7: Rest Day (focusing on relaxation and leisure activities)

Week 2:

Day 8:

Morning: Core Activation and Stability Exercises (15 min)
Afternoon: Dynamic movement sequences for strength and flexibility (20 minutes)
Evening: Progressive Muscle Relaxation for Deeper Body Awareness (10 min)

Day 9:

Morning: Breathing Techniques for Somatic Awareness (10 min)
Afternoon: Body Scan and Grounding Exercises (15 min)
Evening: Spinal Mobility and Alignment Techniques (10 Minutes)

Day 10:

Morning: Functional Movement Patterns for Everyday Activities (20 min)
Afternoon: Integrating Somatics into Cardiovascular Exercise (15 min)
Evening: Mindfulness and Physical Activity (10 minutes)

Day 11:

Morning: Pelvic Floor Engagement and Core Strengthening Exercises (15 Minutes)
Afternoon: Movement Exploration for Body Alignment (20 min)
Evening: Stress Reduction and Relaxation Techniques (10 Minutes)

Day 12:

Morning: Gentle Stretching Routine (10 minutes).
Afternoon: Mindful Eating and Somatic Awareness (15 minutes)
Evening: Restorative Practices and Self-Care (meditation or a hot bath).

Day 13:

Morning: Core Activation and Stability Exercises (15 min)
Afternoon: Dynamic movement sequences for strength and flexibility (20 minutes)
Evening: Progressive Muscle Relaxation for Deeper Body Awareness (10 min)

Day 14:

Morning: Breathing Techniques for Somatic Awareness (10 min)
Afternoon: Body Scan and Grounding Exercises (15 min)

Evening: Reflection and goal-setting for the week ahead (10 minutes)

This two-week somatic exercise program takes a balanced approach to increasing body awareness, relaxation, strength, and flexibility. Adjust the routines as required to accommodate individual tastes and abilities.